REMEMBER THE FUTURE

How to Use Visualization and Mental Images to Program Your Mind for Success

RAZA IMAM

Table of Contents

Get Your FREE Gift #1

Get my 1-page cheat sheet **"60 Seconds of Focus"**

I will show you how to develop __ruthless focus__ so you can:

- SKYROCKET your productivity
- TURBOCHARGE your income
- BOOST your self-confidence
- ANNIHILATE debt

My 1-page cheat sheet will help you do all of this by harnessing the power of __ruthless focus.__

Click the link below to get your free gift:

http://www.5xYourFocus.com

WHY THIS BOOK IS SHORT AND SWEET – NO FLUFF

"Give me a one-page bullet-list of exactly what I should do. That's worth more to me than a stack of books that I have to dig through to get to the good stuff. I may give you 50 bucks for the books. But I'll pay you $5,000 for the one page."

That's a quote from Alwyn Cosgrove, a world-famous strength coach and entrepreneur.

In this short book, we've given you everything you need to know about staying focused and achieving your goals. This book is short, and that's for a reason.

We wanted to give you 100% actionable content, not a bunch of fluff and theory.

Sure we give practical examples to prove our point.

Yes we give you specific action items to do and we explain why.

Of course we tell you exactly how to implement these steps to get the best results.

But we worked **ruthlessly** to keep this book short and sweet.

So remember to **take action!**

WHAT HAPPENED WHEN I GOT FOCUSED

Like most 30-something guys with kids, I have a very busy life. Here's my typical day: An hour-long commute to and from work. Helping my 5 year-old with homework. Giving the kids baths. Putting them to bed. Doing dishes. Hanging out with the wife. And going to bed.

Not to mention the community service and volunteer work that I do, visiting friends and family on the weekends, and religious and spiritual commitments that I have.

Currently, I'm 34 with 3 kids, work a full-time job AND write books.

But it wasn't always like this for me.

For the longest time I wanted to make a side income, in addition to my full-time job.

I tried everything; "creative" real estate, internet marketing, blogging, starting a consulting business, and multi-level marketing.

But nothing ever stuck.

After a while, I learned about search engine optimization and created a fitness blog. It started seeing some success so I decided to take my diet and workouts seriously.

It took a few years to finally figure out how to eat and the exact right workouts to do, but after I got the information down, **I started to focus.**

Well, within a few short months I got these results:

- To become a best-selling author on Amazon twice (_The Science of Getting Ripped_ and _30 Days of Focus_)

- To get a promotion at work (with a **15%** raise)

- To build an online business that makes passive income ($500 to $2500 per month)

- To quadruple the size of my email list (in **just** 3 months)

- To build muscle and get down to 10% body fat (in 3 hours a week while **still** eating my favorite foods)

The results were amazing and I know you can do the same.

Get Your FREE Gift #2

I will also email you my other super-popular videos I use to visualize my goals and get focused:

- 6 Minute Daily Visualization for Goal Achievement

- How to Manifest Your Desires (very powerful visualization)

It takes less than 20 minutes to go through and will help you get focused and prime your subconscious mind for success.

You can get access to all of that AND my **"60 Seconds of Focus"** cheat sheet by going here:

www.5xYourFocus.com

WHAT IS THE MENTAL MOVIE METHOD?

Michael Phelps is the all-time record holder in the Olympics. Nobody can even come close. When it comes to gold medal wins or just personal medal count, Michael Phelps is the all-time record holder. A lot of sports commentators marvel at his swimming skills. He is no ordinary Olympic swimmer. A lot of commentators are so amazed by his ability that a lot of them think jokingly that he is part dolphin.

As successful as Michael Phelps may be, his success wasn't inborn. There are many other athletes out there with better physiques. There are many other competitors out there that have bodies that are better suited for the water. It's not like his success is genetically predetermined.

The bottom line is he wasn't simply handed his medals because of the random luck of his genetics. Instead, he overcame tough competition from all four corners of the world to win each and every one of his medals. He earned his success. How? He trained. And trained. And trained. End of story. Michael Phelps's victory is earned victory. Nobody handed it to him. He didn't have it in the bag by virtue of being born in the right place or at the right time. It's all about training.

Now, this opens another set or inquiry because let's face it, if it's just training, then there are other competitors out there that trained as hard as Michael Phelps and, some would argue, even harder. As rigorous as Phelps's training may have been, other athletes also trained. How come he achieved better results than other competitors who may have even trained harder than him?

Phelps had a secret weapon: the mental movie system. This book unpacks this secret system so you yourself can benefit from it. The great news is that the mental movie system is not custom made for Micheal Phelps. It worked tremendously for him, but you could also make it to work for you.

Whether you are trying to do better at school, at work, or in your relationships, or you are trying to find the willpower and motivation to hit the gym and develop the best body you can achieve, the mental movie system will work for you. Again, it is not unique to Michael Phelps. It is not custom-made for him. Instead, it works with all people from all walks of life, in all areas of the world. Put simply, if the mental movie success system can work for Michael Phelps, it can work for you as well. If he can do it, you can too. This book steps you through the process of having this powerful and almost unstoppable system work to your personal advantage.

THE 2 MOST DEBILITATING MYTHS ABOUT SUCCESS

Before we get to how the mental movie system works and how you can use it, let's just get one thing out of the way. There are lots of commonly held beliefs that sabotage success. If you subscribe to any of these common beliefs, your ability to achieve success in your life will be greatly stymied. Make sure that you understand what these myths are, and make sure that you do not believe them.

I can't emphasize this enough: what you believe, you will achieve. It's easy to understand this in a positive way. If you believe something is possible, you are more likely to achieve that particular objective or outcome. But it also works in a negative way. If you believe that certain things are not possible or if you have certain limiting beliefs, then your ability to achieve success will be greatly reduced.

It all boils down to what you choose to believe. And unfortunately, there are lots of myths and misconceptions out there that sabotage people's ability to succeed. The worst part of all of this is that they try really hard. It's not like they're lazy. It's not like they don't put in the effort and time to try to achieve success. Unfortunately, their own beliefs end up sabotaging and undermining them.

You have to be clear regarding these two common myths. Otherwise, you are going to fail. There is really no way around it. You are just setting yourself up for disappointment.

Myth #1: You Only Need to Train to Be Successful

This thinking assumes that people who already know what to do will be successful. They believe that if you do the right training and do the right process and pick up the right skills and have the right talent, you will be successful.

At first glance, this seems perfectly reasonable. After all, how many times can you pack the word "right" in the idea above? Unfortunately, this is not true. There are many highly skilled, highly talented people who always come in at number two. And that's assuming they rank at all.

Make no mistake about it. When Michael Phelps competes in an Olympic pool, the people around him are not slackers. They are people who put in long hours of rigorous training. In fact, some of them probably worked harder at training than Michael Phelps. They go out of their way to go through the right training process to pick up the right skills and hone the right talents, but success still evades them. Sure, they can come close, but you and I know that when it comes to the competition of life, you have to shoot for number one. They come in at number two, and that's assuming they come in at all.

The bottom line is undeniable: while knowing what to do is important, it doesn't adequately explain why some people seem to win all the time while others who are similarly talented can't seem to get a break. These similarly talented people work just as hard, if not more. There must be something else. They're going through the right training, they're developing the right skill sets, and they seem to have the right set of talents, but they can't seem to come in at number one on a predictable basis.

Myth #2: It's All About Luck

The other end of the extreme is another equally seductive explanation. If you think about it hard enough, these two myths are actually joined at the hip. Imagine yourself as a person who is working to with the right training system and trying to build up the right skills and pick up the right talents. You're just going through the proper checklist that everybody says will lead to success. You put in the work. You know you put in the time. Still, you can't come in at number one regularly. In fact, if you come in at all, you come in at number two.

It's very tempting to believe that after you have put in all the time, effort, energy, and emotional investment to come in at the top and fail to do that, that it must be all about luck. According to this thinking, you should eventually just focus less on having the right stuff. Instead, focus on just knowing enough about what you're doing so that when opportunity appears, you can be at the right place at the right time.

This is very seductive and appealing to many people because of its primary premise involving effort. This common myth can actually be used to excuse yourself from having to train as hard. Since in the back of your head, you're thinking that regardless of how intense your training is, it all boils down to luck. So why should you train as hard? Do you see how this works? It is no surprise that a lot of athletes actually believe this, regardless of how hard they train on the surface.

The good news is that this is also false. You have to put in the work. You have to go through the process. You can't just focus on "doing enough".

As tempting as the concept of luck may be, if you want to achieve predictable and sustainable success, you have to focus on putting in the work. You have to train really hard. You have to invest the proper amount of time, effort, and energy in whatever you're doing. The old saying, "The harder I work, the luckier I get," is 100% true. Why? The more time and effort you put into what you're doing, the easier it would be to spot opportunities. This is the real deal.

The myth is that you just need to do enough so you would spot opportunities. That's not true. You have to train really hard and repeat the same process over and over again, and often work from many different perspectives and avenues so you can be able to spot opportunities properly. Does this mean that if you just slack off, that you wouldn't be able to spot opportunities? Absolutely not. You may be able to do that, but if you want to develop this skill so that it predictably works for you, you need to put in the work.

Success is all about spotting opportunities and taking advantage of them. When you work really hard at training or some sort of preparation for a career, or doing the job that you're already doing, you invest in your ability to spot opportunities. You also invest in others' perceptions of you. When they perceive that you have put in the time, then they are more likely to believe that you are more qualified. This opens doors of opportunities.

Make no mistake about it. Opportunities don't magically appear. They are already there. It just takes work and preparation to spot them or to be viewed as qualifies for them.

The Bottom Line

If you believe any of these myths or variations of them, understand that they rob you of your success. They give you all sorts of excuses to not try as hard. They also set up all sorts of expectations that ultimately lead to defeat.

For example, if you believe in the first myth that you only need to train really hard and things will fall into place, then it only takes a few defeats to rob you of your passion. You feel that you're just banging your head against a wall and you are tempted to just give up.

Remember, you will only fail if you quit. Unfortunately, you may feel so discouraged and so emotionally tapped out because your assumptions had set up the wrong expectations. You end up giving up. There are no two ways about it. These two myths and their many, many variations serve to rob you of your success. Make sure that you don't believe them.

SUCCESS IS SPECIFIC

The essence of success is all about process. It's all about going through the proper steps, and then focusing. This is not a simple matter of going through the right training. I mean, you can train as much as you want, but you have to come up with a specific process based on your own set of experiences and your own set of particular circumstances. There is no one-size-fits-all or cookie cutter approach to success. While there are basic templates that can be used as starting points, that's all they are: starting points. You have to understand that hitting the gym, swimming many laps in the pool, or running several miles a day is just the template. They do not, in and of themselves, guarantee success. Instead, you have to train in such a way that you focus on your specific reality.

Priming Yourself for Competition Using Your Specific Reality

As I mentioned above, simply going through physical exercises is just the first step. Putting in the effort is just the launching point. The process that you're getting into should actually be customized for yourself.

To prime yourself for success, you have to look at each competition as a unique event. Each is dynamic. While you can train to give yourself a template for success, it is just a starting point. Each competition has its own dynamic reality. This reality changes from situation to situation. And each competition is a product of a specific moment.

If you're able to understand this, then you would be in the right place to do what's needed for however long to achieve success for that particular competition, project, trial, or obstacle.

Success Is Not Abstract, but Rooted in a Specific Point in Reality

This is what many people miss. They think that success is really just all about filling in all the blanks. If they put in X number of hours, they go through X number of credits in college, or meet X person, they would be successful.

It doesn't work that way for most people. If you want predictable success, understand that it is rooted in a specific point in reality. Success is specific. It's specific in time, it has a specific place, it takes a specific form.

One of the most common ways to view this is that you're competing against specific people with their own particular sets of strengths and weaknesses. In other words, you're dealing with something dynamic, and this is why a lot of other "success systems" out there fail and fail again. They may have worked for the person who came up with the system because of his or her specific set of circumstances. I can guarantee that those circumstances may not apply to you. When you implement their system, chances are you'll fall flat on your face. Which brings up my next point.

Most People Prepare for Success in the Abstract

When you are simply filling in the blanks or following some sort of checklist or you're implementing some sort of success framework, you're just shooting for success in the abstract. You prepare in general or you use broad tools.

As I mentioned above, you may be using tools or systems that may have been implemented by somebody with a particular set of circumstances that might not apply to you. They might not apply to the situation that you're trying to apply them to. They just focus on the tools that you have, and then they don't focus on the specifics of what you will do at that specific time. Not surprisingly, these systems produce hit or miss success.

Now, don't get me wrong. I'm not saying that they completely fail all the time. I will never say that. What I am saying is that they're not going to give you what you're looking for, which is predictable success. How can they? They produce hit or miss success.

Things work out this way because if enough of your "general picture" fits the reality of your situation, you will succeed. In other words, if your particular situation fits the ideal environment, settings, or assumptions behind the success system you're trying to implement, then you have a higher chance of succeeding. If, on the other hand, you leave off too much or there is a lot of ambiguities, or the situation you're trying to impose the system on is simply just too incompatible, you're not going to get what you need to get. The general idea that you have of what you need to do, when you need to do it, simply won't fit. An important element might be left missing, and you end up failing.

So what are these common "hit or miss" strategies?

Common Faulty Strategies

Here are just some of the personal success strategies out there. They apply to people who are trying to get fit, lose weight, get better jobs, or achieve greater happiness and personal power. Whatever you're trying to achieve, there are many personal development books out there, but they all fall into three distinct caps.

Now, I'm not going to pretend that all the categories below pretty much sums up all the self-help books out there. I'm not going to say that. What I am going to say is that these are great starting points for the bulk of the materials out there. There are many other categories. But I list these to give you a general idea of what common strategies exist, and why they fall flat.

Give It 110%

One common approach is to just go in there with both barrels blazing and just mow down everything that gets in your way. As the old saying goes, the best defense is a great offense. So you just go in there and use a "shock and awe" approach.

This all sounds great in theory, but if you look closely enough to what you actually do, it falls flat. What if the specific situation requires none of the other parts of what you've trained for? In other words, you come in with a script of what you're supposed to do. But when the competition comes, it turned out that the specific situation requires none of the other parts that you have practiced, and used only one particular part. Unfortunately, you did not emphasize that part enough. You're looking at the broad picture, so you focus on everything else.

For example, you're going to take the bar exam to become an attorney and there are many different subjects that you have to study. And the bar exam actually featured a part that you did not study enough for. You studied it, but you glossed it over because there are many other parts that need to be covered. What if that happens? This also applies to athletic competitions. For example, you may have anticipated that certain parts of a trail will require more effort, but it turns out that the actual conditions on the ground were much different from your assumptions.

When you try to give something 110%, you eventually end up spreading yourself too thin. You either over-rehearse and over-prepare, or you do the complete opposite. Things don't really pan out the way you would expect if you use such a broad template as just simply giving an activity more effort than usual.

Just Prepare to Work Hard

Working hard is good. Let's get that out of the way. There's nothing wrong with working hard. However, if you're not working specifically for that particular objective that you have in front of you, or preparing for that specific competition in front of you, then your efforts would be hit or miss. It will be too little, too late. Working hard is great, but it's not enough by itself.

Attitude Is Everything

Another commonly held success strategy is that as long as you work on your attitude, everything else will fall into place. I wish this was true. I wish it were true that you just need to think the right thoughts and you will somehow magically "attract" the right results.

Well, you can think all fantastic and amazing things that you want sitting down, but unless you take sustained action, nothing's going to happen. This is like me imagining myself being ripped like Arnold Schwarzenegger. But when I'm thinking, I'm sitting on my chair eating Cheetos and drinking beer. It doesn't matter how vivid the images are in my mind, and it doesn't matter how palpable my "winning attitude" may be. I'm not going to lose that spare tire around my gut. It's simply not going to happen.

Attitude without action is worthless. Even if you were to take action, you still have to take the right action for the right moment and in the right context. If you just "do it", you might end up doing the wrong thing, or you might be thinking too generally and do something that doesn't really fit the particular situation you're in.

I can't emphasize this enough. Success is not some sort of abstract framework. It's rooted in a specific point in reality. It's specific in time, place, form, and yes, personnel.

Unless you're able to wrap your mind around this and focus on the variables involved, even your very best efforts are not going to be enough. You may have the best attitude in the world, you may be bringing in 110%, but you will eventually fall short more often than not. Now, this doesn't mean that those techniques don't produce success from time to time. They do, but if you're looking for something more than just a hit or miss approach to greater personal success and effectiveness, you need to keep reading. Thankfully, there is a better alternative.

WANT TO SUPERCHARGE YOUR RESULTS?

I will show you how to develop **ruthless focus** so you can:

- SKYROCKET your productivity
- TURBOCHARGE your income
- BOOST your self-confidence
- ANNIHILATE debt

My 1-page cheat sheet will help you do all of this by harnessing the power of **ruthless focus**

I will also email you my other super-popular videos I use to visualize my goals and get focused:

- 6 Minute Daily Visualization for Goal Achievement
- How to Manifest Your Desires (very powerful visualization)

They take less than 20 minutes to go through and will help you get focused and prime your subconscious mind for success.

You can get access to all of that by going here:

<u>www.5xYourFocus.com</u>

Go there now to get the 1-page cheat sheet and these great videos.

Here's that link again: <u>www.5xYourFocus.com</u>

FAILURE HAPPENS

What if your best isn't good enough? What if you went through the checklist, made sure that everything was in place and you did everything the right way? Or so you thought.

Well, I've got some bad news for you. Even if you went through your list several times over, you can still fail. Even if you gave it 110% or even 1000%, you can still fail. Finally, even if you have the best attitude on the planet, you can still fail.

Failure happens. Get over it. This is reality. And this is exactly why most people fail. They have a very warped or unrealistic view of failure. Let me get something clear about failure so you can use the mental movie method to produce sustainable success.

Again, we're not talking about hitting the mark once in a while. We're not talking about coming in first sporadically. Anybody can do that, seriously. If you just follow all the other success books on the market out there, you can achieve sporadic success. I suspect that you are reading this book because you are tired of sporadic success. You're tired of hoping that somehow, somewhere, everything lands up and you sneak into first place. Well, that's not predictable success. That's not performing at your peak level. That's not living your life to its highest level of victory. If you want to achieve all of that, then you need to first start with a realistic view of success.

Failure Happens Even If...

Failure happens even if you're prepared, okay? Let's just get that out of the way. Even if you put in 110% or you outworked everybody and you made sure that everything is planned out properly, you can still fail. Failure happens even if you worked hard.

This is very heartbreaking for most people because this reality really flies in the face of how most people view success in life. The standard view is if you put in the time, effort, energy, and made the right sacrifices, you will succeed.

There is no doubt about that. You will succeed, but it's going to be success that is sporadic. That's not enough. Working hard can get you 80% of the way, but it doesn't guarantee predictable, consistent, and constant success. Do you want to win almost all the time? Or do you want to win from time to time? Do you want to win just because somebody dropped the ball or because somebody failed to show up at the right time?

If you are settling for sporadic success, I've got some bad news for you. Almost everybody is capable of sporadic success. If you're looking to win in dribs and drabs, you just need to focus on working hard. That will get you there.

But if you're reading this book because you are sick and tired of success being "drip-fed" into your life, then you have to wrap your mind around the central fact that failure happens even if you worked hard. To make matters worse, failure happens even if you thought your project out. That's right, even if you resolve to work smart instead of just hard, victory can still slip through your fingers.

You have to understand that when people think through their project, they're usually thinking in abstract terms. They're not looking at the specific moment, nor are they looking to create a specific moment. They're just looking at the project in terms of an overview. It's like some sort of template that they would apply to all sorts of projects, regardless of the specific details of the projects. That's not good enough. Now, mind you, that it will get you 80-90% of the way to victory, but it's not enough to clinch the title. It's not enough to get through the goal line. Do you see how this works?

Which brings to mind the next point. Even if you have a good attitude, failure happens. Even if you have an invincible attitude, failure will still happen. Attitude is really important. Don't get me wrong. As the old saying goes, your attitude determines your altitude. Your attitude enables you to find the focus, passion, and energy needed to keep pounding away until you achieve a breakthrough. Your attitude also dictates the amount of passion and energy you need so you can constantly scale up what you're doing.

A good attitude is indispensable for success, but in and of itself, it's not going t o take you there. It's not enough. There are lots of people all over this planet who have tremendous attitudes who can withstand the most heart-crushing disaster, but they're struggling. Which brings up the final point here: even if you're motivated, failure can still happen.

Motivation is not enough. You have to have the right system, as well. You have to be motivated enough to pay attention to the right details at a specific point in time to achieve victory in that present time at that present place.

You see how specific this is? Do you see how the specificity of victory essentially escapes all the feel good generalizations and "one size fits all" success frameworks out there. You have to come up with a blueprint.

31

TAKE CONTROL - FAILURE IS NOT FATAL

Now that we have some very important, although painful, truths out of the way, now let's focus on the ultimate reality of failure. Why does failure happen? Why do otherwise well-prepared, highly trained, and highly motivated people with the best attitudes in the world fall short?

It's very simple. It all boils down to mental failure at a specific place and at a specific time. If you were to take that person out of that very specific place in time, they can do really well in theory. They can do really well in other types of context, but unfortunately they drop the ball at that point in time. They screwed up at that particular place.

It all boils down to mental failure. You fail to see ahead what could go wrong and prepare for them in the moment. You can theoretically prepare, but you have to be ready at the moment.

You also fail to fit what you're doing with what you should be doing, based on the actual conditions as they play out. This happens all the time, whether we're talking about the stock trading floor, the football field, the baseball diamond, the Olympic swimming pool, you name it. People fail because of mental failure. In most cases, it has nothing to do with their physical state. It has nothing to do with being big enough, having the right background, having put enough money in their training. In most cases, it's about mental failure.

Ultimately, failure and success boils down to whether your failure is less than the failure of your competitors. This is what so many other self-help and self-development completely overlook. They trick you into thinking that life's competitions and struggles essentially involve this flat, featureless, generic landscape where the competitors are always the same and the conditions don't change.

Nothing could be further from the truth. You only need to look at the NBA. Why do you think Michael Jordan and the Chicago Bulls were unstoppable? It's because their other competitors were not at their peak at that specific point in time. Do you see how this works? The same could be said of the New England Patriots, the LA Lakers, with Magic, and then with Kobe. The same could be said with the Boston Celtics, with Larry Bird. It's not enough for the participants to be at the top of their game, but they also have to perform at such a level that it beats the failure rate of their competitors. In fact, even a fast-rising team like Philadelphia 76ers with Allen Iverson, who is such a phenomenal player, they can only go so far because it's all comparative. It doesn't matter how talented the person is and how much time, effort, and energy they put into it. Unless their failure level is less than the failure of their competitors, they will lose.

Most other self-improvement books completely overlook this or try to hide this fact. They try to look at the problem from a completely different perspective and that's why people get the wrong impression, why people are laboring under false assumptions. But it really all boils down to that.

Once again, failure and success boils down to whether your failure at a specific place and a specific time is less than the failure of your competitors. This is how success works.

Unfortunately, this is not enough. If you're going to compete in such a way where you're just hoping that your failure rate is less than the failure rate of your competitors, then you are just hoping to get lucky. That's the bottom line. This is the wrong way to compete, because you're essentially just hoping that Lady Luck shines your way. You are hoping against hope that you are lucky enough to be paired with substandard competitors. It's like there Roger Federer hoping that

Rafael Nadal has a cold right before their match. You can't bank on your competitors performing at a substandard level. You can't bank on your competitors feeling under the weather. It just doesn't work.

This is why the general approach of most other self-development books fall flat. They sound great, they get you excited, but really, it all boils down to either avoiding, ignoring, overlooking, or deceptively working with the fact that failure and success boils down to whether your failure is less than the failure of your competitors. This is not the way forward. There has to be a better way.

Inconsistent Failure Leads to Unstable Success

Since most people approach their personal quest for success using the standard concept mentioned above, then it's no surprise that most people's experience with success is quite erratic and unstable. It all boils down to you win some, you lose some. Sometimes, your competitors really outshine you because they're just at the top of their game at that time and your failure level is higher than them. So you end up losing. Sometimes, you fail slightly less than them, and you come out ahead. You're essentially just banking on others being weak so you can win. What if you come across someone who's strong almost all the time? What happens then? Well, you know the answer.

Another reason why this approach and almost all other approaches fail is because you're banking on all parameters of a situation being just right. You're also hoping that your preparation is enough, compared to others. In other words, your preparation covered enough of the circumstances and operational parameters of the competition so you come out ahead. That is assuming too much. It's not going to pan out. Not by a long shot.

The Truth: Success Is Specific

You have to look at success without generalization. You have to look at success without some of the comforting lies of most "success programs".

The truth is that success is specific. It has a specific time, a specific context, and you will be up against specific competitors with their own particular range of strengths and weaknesses. There is no one-size-fits-all solution.

A real solution must factor in this specificity. Otherwise, you're just hoping against hope that your badly-fitting strategy produces enough results that slightly edges everybody else in the competition. That is too much to hope for. You can't bank on that happening. Thankfully, there is an alternative.

The Secret to CONSISTENT Victory: Total Control Over Your Situation

Make no mistake about it. You have a lot more control over your life than you give yourself credit for.

The reason why you have this tremendous amount of control is you're always perceiving reality and judging otherwise neutral data points your body is picking up. This is how you edit your reality. Make no mistake about it. When you think about something, you are engaged in judgment. You are giving it meaning. This is how you edit your reality.

Two people can look at the exact same situation. It doesn't matter whether it's a building burning down, people getting shot at, earthquakes, you name it. But those people can respond to the situation in two totally different ways. You can respond by freaking out and giving in to your emotions, and end up achieving very little in terms of productive outcomes, or you can respond calmly so you can preserve assets, maintain relative calm, and eventually weather what would otherwise be a traumatic situation.

It all boils down to your response. So I need you to direct your attention to this central reality, because you have that power. Nobody can take that away from you except yourself. You have to assert total control over your situation when you're competing. That's the only thing you can control.

When you control your mindset, you control your emotions. When you control your emotions, you control your body and your actions. When you control your actions, you control how people perceive you.

It all begins with your frame of mind. Everything else is a non-option. You can't control your competitors and their skill levels. Some people are just more skilled than you. You can work on boosting up your skills, but they can level up and catch up, and even surpass you. You can't control them. You definitely can't control your location. If your boss says to show up to give a sales talk at a particular place, you're going to show up. It's not like you can say, "Yeah, I'd like to have the venue moved." Sometimes it happens, but you can't bank on that.

You also can't control the natural factors surrounding the competition or event. Maybe it would be raining. Maybe there was a flu outbreak and people are feeling under the weather. All sorts of things can happen in terms of the natural world. You can't control that. Finally, you can't control random events. Remember, Murphy's Law is always in effect. It seems like the worst thing that can possibly happen almost always happens at the worst time. That's just how the cookie crumbles.

But the good news despite all of this uncertainty is that you have a lot more control over what's happening in your life and how you choose to perceive and respond to reality than you give yourself credit for.

MASTER YOUR MINDSET

Before I start laying out the specifics of the mental movie method, let me just establish the proper foundation for the solution. You have to go through this. You have to have a clear understanding of how this works so you can straighten up what you need to straighten up. You can let go of certain limiting beliefs, you might want to forget about certain limiting assumptions that you may have subscribed to. It all boils down to your mindset.

How You Choose to Perceive a Situation Leads to Control

Have you ever wondered why otherwise well-prepared and highly-skilled and talented people choke in the worst way possible? It's not like they lack training. It's not like they're not talented. But for some reason or other, they choke. They fumble the pass, they say the wrong things at a sales call, they misread messages, and they don't get the date. What do these all have in common?

It all boils down to perception. They perceive the situation in a way that they lose control. At the very least, they perceive a situation in a way that they're no longer in a position to respond in an optimal way.

For example, if you're normally a decent basketball player. You might be thinking, "I'm going to play ball and I'm going to win." You approach the situation very confidently, you prepare yourself. And then when you show up, the person is incredibly talented and you can't help but feel inferior. Your game is thrown off and you can barely make a basket. You don't exactly make an amazing first impression.

The issue here is not whether you're prepared or not. The issue is not whether you're good or not. It has nothing to do with any of those. What it has to do is how you chose to perceive a situation. You look at the external stimuli of this person being better than you expected, and it threw you off. You feel that, "I'm better than this guy, but why can't I make a shot?" There's thousands of these types of thoughts going through your mind, and the end result is all too predictable. You lost control. It all boils down to how you perceive the situation.

Now, can you imagine if you looked at that person and chose to perceive him or her the same way as the typical person that you normally play against? If that's your mindset, then you wouldn't make a fool out of yourself. You would have a much higher chance of winning. Do you see how this works?

The best part of all of this is that you can choose to perceive a situation a certain way. You're always in command. You're always in the driver's seat. So choose to perceive a situation that leads to greater control, instead of lower control.

We May Not Be the Cause, But We Control How We Respond

I want you to go back to what I said earlier regarding two people looking at a burning building or people getting shot. We may not have caused the building to burn down, we may not have pulled the trigger that killed people and caused mayhem, but we can always control how we respond.

How we choose to respond is extremely important because the world judges us by our actions. I just want to make it clear that the world couldn't care less what your intentions or motivations are. The world couldn't care less about what you would have, should have, or could have done. All it cares about is what you actually did or failed to do. That's the bottom line. This is called objective reality.

We're judged by our actions. I mean, we can talk a big game regarding what motivates us or our intentions. We can paint flowery pictures of our hopes, dreams, and motivations, but ultimately, it really all boils down to objective reality. What did you do?

I need you to keep coming back to this central fact, because you may not be the cause of the disasters happening in your life, but you can control how you respond. That's how you control the outcome.

What happens when you step up? You start taking control when you step up and take control of your life. You end up sticking to the script. The script is very simple. It's what you're supposed to do in a particular situation. It reminds you of your range of options at a particular point in time. You are then clear on how you should respond to changes that deviate from the script.

If you keep repeating the script many times and then playing off many different variations, a contingency plan of action quickly comes to mind. If you're able to see how the contingency plan grows from this standard script, then it's going to be very hard for you to be thrown off. Regardless of the particular shape that the competition, the challenge, or the trial takes, it's very hard to throw you off because you already know what you're supposed to do, and you also prepared for what could go wrong, and your contingency plan of action.

Even if you haven't fully mapped out all the specific contingencies, simply having contingency plans in place puts you in a much better position than your competitors.

So what's the result if you do this? You will remain calm. In any kind of challenge, the situations can always quickly veer from ideal to less than ideal. While your competitors were thrown off, you remain calm. Again, going back to the burning building analogy, while another person sees a burning building and promptly proceeds to freak out and start running around like a chicken with its head cut off, you remain calm. You don't get thrown off. You end up with a tremendous sense of opportunity. You are in a better position to do the right thing, to ensure a better resolution.

Also, when you stick to the script and are aware of contingency plans, you remain focused on the reward. You don't freak out about what you're going to lose. You don't freak out and get desperate. You don't overreact because you feel that this gorgeous person is never going to call you again.

Put simply, feeling that things are wrong or have gone down the toilet aren't going to throw you off track. Finally, you begin to think and move in a routine manner. If you understand all these, then you would see how somebody that's able to pull this off again and again and again in particular specific situations and contexts would be more successful than others.

Solutions to Attaining the Proper Success Mindset

As I mentioned earlier, to achieve success with a mental movie method, you really have to focus on your mindset. To prepare, you have to use tried and proven techniques that would enable you to better tap the raw power of your mind.

You can pick any of the techniques below. I'm not saying one is necessarily better than the other. I'm giving you a choice of three, although there are many others out there. I just believe that these three are the most attainable and most accessible approaches. Feel free to customize them based on your personal preference, needs, or background.

Technique #1: Meditation/Mindfulness

Meditation and mindfulness are becoming really popular nowadays in the United States and Western Europe. They've been around for thousands of years in the East. In the Western philosophical and spiritual tradition, they've also been around, but in different forms.

Regardless of the "flavor" of meditation and mindfulness you're interested in, they all share one particular quality: then enable you to focus on the present moment. This is how you know you're dealing with a legitimate mindfulness or meditation practice. Without this element, you're not engaged in meditation and mindfulness. You really aren't. Because this is the lowest common denominator of all the many different flavors, traditions, and practices out there. It's all about focusing on the present moment. You learn to train your mind where you are at a specific point in time.

Advantages

The big advantage of meditation and mindfulness is that they help you focus on the moment, which enables you to divorce emotions from thoughts. The reason why a lot of people get thrown off their best game is because when certain thoughts come to mind, they respond in a negative way. They get all emotional and they get thrown off track.

If you practice meditation or mindfulness enough, you would be able to reach a point where you can separate the judgment from your thought. At the very least, your thoughts would be neutral. This enables you to achieve a state of equal-mindedness or equanimity.

This is very important because it triggers mental peace that would enable you to do what's right at the right time and at the right place. This is precisely what you need if you are in a competition. As the competition heats up and there's certain dynamic in the game, you have to know what the next step is. You have to zero in on the proper course of action. This is hard to do if you are operating out of fear, annoyance, irritation, or you're letting your physical exhaustion get the best of you.

Disadvantages

The big disadvantage of meditation and mindfulness for many people in the West is that in many cases, it gets too deep. You just want the ability to divorce your emotion from your thoughts. You just want the ability to stay in the moment. However, depending on the particular meditation practice, you can learn about chakras and unleashing certain negative energy. While this can be very positive, they also take time. You might get distracted.

Also, there are many flavors on mindfulness and meditation. This could lead to confusion.

Another drawback is that these techniques may be too broad for you. Make no mistake about it. They help you build some sort of mental discipline. That's indisputable. But the problem is it may not be specific enough to what you need to do at a specific point of time and place. In other words, it may not be enough for you to use in a competition. The good news is that as long as you keep practicing and fine-tuning your mindfulness practice, you will be able to unleash its benefits and free yourself from its disadvantages.

However, this also brings to mind another negative, which is it requires constant practice. There are no two ways about it. Mindfulness and meditation is not much different from going to the gym. At the gym, you work out your body. You try to build up your muscles. When you meditate and practice mindfulness, you work out your mental and emotional muscles. Just like muscles, if you don't work out for a long enough period of time, or you work out very sporadically, your muscles begin to shrink and they become weaker and weaker.

The same applies to mindfulness and meditation. This could be a problem if you're like the typical busy American. Time is a luxury for many people, and you might not be able to find the 10-20 minutes you need everyday to practice mindfulness.

Technique #2: Constant Practice

Another approach you could take is to constantly practice. You're just looking at the task that you're supposed to do and really blowing it up. You're looking at it from many different perspectives, you're analyzing all the aspects, and then you train in them. You work at mastering both the form and the substance. You not only figure out what to do and how to do it, but you also have a clear understanding of why certain aspects and elements are required by or are present in your project.

The big advantage here is with constant practice, you master the many different aspects of the task, which leads to the biggest advantage of a sense of ease. You're no longer stressed out. You no longer feel that this is going to be a hassle. You start looking forward to it. In fact, you get really excited about the competition or the project. This sense of ease enables you to take the right action at the right time.

Disadvantages

Constant practice is great, but it suffers from a very debilitating weakness: it is not rooted in a specific time, place, or context. When you practice, you're just essentially hoping that the ideal conditions are as you imagined them to be. Alternatively, you are hoping that the assumptions that you are making in the context of your practice remain the same. This is too much to ask. As a result, you may not be able to anticipate problems.

Also, you might be fuzzy on specific forms of victory. You might be training "just to win". Well, just to win isn't enough. In sports competition, victory takes a specific shape. In many other activities, ultimate victory takes a specific shape. Constant practice has a broad definition of the success you're trying to achieve.

Again, don't get me wrong. While constant practice can get you 80-90% of the way, it doesn't deliver 100%. It can't. It can't account for variations. It can't account for contingencies that seem to pop out of nowhere. Ultimately, they may not be broad enough. Constant training may not be broad enough to tackle things that may go wrong.

Technique #3: Modeling

Modeling is all about tapping the power of "monkey see, monkey do." The idea here is if you copy what successful people do in particular situations, you achieve what they achieve. Very simple, very basic, and also very powerful.

The big advantage here is you get motivated, seriously. You unleash a tremendous wave of motivation because nothing gets people striving for success more excited than seeing the actual success of people who are trying to do what they're trying to achieve. It doesn't get any more basic than that.

You get to look at an actual track record of success. This is documented, this is proven. This is not just a case of somebody saying that their uncle achieved something.

You can break things up, you can slice and dice the facts. It's real. This is objective reality.

Since this speaks to the rational side of your mind, you can then use them as case studies to get a positive emotional payoff. You would be able to constantly refer back to that role model who achieved success and tap into a sense of possibility. Again, it all boils down to realizing that if they can do it, you can do it, too.

Of course, this assumes that there's really nothing fundamentally different between you and your role model. You have to suspend your disbelief, at least in this particular instance. You can't model yourself after somebody who made a billion dollars because his father left him 900 million dollars. It won't work if you don't have 900 million dollars lying around. Do you see how this works? So there has to be some assumptions there that by and large, you have the same resources or you're dealing with the same challenges and that your cases are similar enough for you to benefit from the model provided by the person you're focused on.

Disadvantages

The big disadvantage here is that a lot of role models may have written their biographies in a selective way. They might not be telling you important details. They might not be telling you that they already have a leg up or they have some sort of advantage. Also, you can't get into their heads and see what really drives them forward.

For example, you may be motivated by the story of Steve Jobs. Steve Jobs was given up for adoption at birth. He was a hippie and dropped out of college after one semester. A lot of people thought he was a dreamer and essentially is going to end up a loser. Boy, did he surprise everybody in his community, and the world for that matter, because he became a billionaire many times over. If that isn't impressive enough, he also changed the world. He changed the way people looked at and developed a relationship with their technology.

As impressive as this narrative is, it's assuming too much that this narrative is accurate, as far as Steve Jobs' internal motivations go. This is a serious impediment to achieving the right mindset through modeling, because ultimately you are trying to pattern your mindset against things that you assume are real, or are reported to be real. But ultimately, you can't get into the head of your model. Your role model may appear to you as a paragon of resilience, tenacity, and imagination, but if you were to take a peek into their heart, they may actually be completely different people. Understand this limitation.

Finally, keep in mind that using role models for mindset building is limited by the fact that you can only look at your role model's success in broad terms. You just hope that you're motivated enough by their success that you can fit it into your specific situation. This is too much to assume, because as inspiring as Steve Jobs may be, he lived in a particular place in a particular time frame. The specific situation you may find yourself in may not necessarily fit into a situation so neatly for you to get all the technical guidance you need. Instead, you are left with looking at your role model's life as a source of broad guidance.

When trying to get your mindset in the right place, try out all the three approaches above. Pick the approach that best fits your particular situation, preference, and needs.

THE BETTER SOLUTION
THE MENTAL MOVIE METHOD

What do all movies have in common? If you've had your share of movie watching, you would know that you can see them at your convenience. You just pop in the DVD or load the file on your computer or tablet, and you're watching a movie. It's very convenient to watch movies unless you're going to watch one that is still in its theatrical release. However, outside of watching movies that are currently in the cinema, you can pretty much watch movies at your convenience.

In terms of content, movies can be very vivid. In fact, this is the hallmark of truly great movies. Worthless movies are those that don't withstand the test of time aren't very vivid. It's obvious that you're watching a movie. There's some sort of "divide" between you and the entertainment that you're watching.

Classic movies are a spring to life. It feels like you are riveted to what's happening on the screen in front of you. This is because great movies are emotionally engaging;

they hit hot buttons. You can't help but be invested in what you're watching emotionally.

Another common feature of all movies is that there's always the same. I don't mean that they all have the same actors and plots. I'm not talking about the content at all. Instead, I'm talking about the fact that the movie is not going to change once it's released on DVD. The movie that you see is going to be the same regardless of how many times you play that DVD or that .mp4 file. It's locked in; it always has the same content. It never changes.

Another important feature of movies is that you feel you have control over them. When you watch the movie repeatedly, you don't feel that it throws you off because you've seen it before. You already understand the plot and how it works. This gives you a sense of control. You can anticipate what's going to happen next. This is because the more you watch movies, the more details you see.

I remember when I first watched The Godfather I and II series. There's still a lot of debate, whether Godfather 3 was a good movie or not, but we can pretty much all universally agree that Godfather I and II are quite significant. I can't help but watch these movies over and over again. Every time I watch them, I pick up new details. I pick up interesting dynamics between the characters. I notice details regarding the plot lines and their implications.

Finally, with repeated viewing of movies, you feel so familiar with the material that you can anticipate each scene. It can get to the point where you anticipate alternate plot twists or actions in the movie. This is really important to note. These alternate plot twists and actions do not actually take place in the movie. Instead, you watch the movie over and over again that you can anticipate how it moves and in your mind, you can come up with alternative twists and turns that the movie could take.

I've reviewed with you the qualities of typical movies because I want you to be clear as to these common features and how they can help you achieve a much higher level of personal productivity, effectiveness, power, and ultimately, success.

The Michael Phelps method IS the mental movie method

Make no mistake about it. In interview after interview with Michael Phelps and his coach, one thing stands out. He is using a version of the mental movie method. His coach taught him to play a mental videotape; this is before and after his training sessions. He sees himself assume a certain posture; he looks at his surroundings, and then he sees himself swimming through the water in a particular way.

When he does this, everything flows according to plan. There's a script that he is following in the movie. In this movie, all the details are clear. Ultimately, it ends at the moment of victory. I would add that after playing this movie repeatedly, he anticipates what could go wrong and how to fix them.

In the same way you watch a movie, you see each scene make way to another scene, and then the plot takes twists and turns. With repeated viewing, you can come up with your own alternative twists and actions. Now this is not what you see in the movie, but this can play out in your mind. You keep watching the movie, and you ask yourself, "What would have happened if Fredo in the Godfather said this to Michael?" or "What would have happened if Sonny did not get killed?" Do you see how this works? You already know the characters and the plot twists in the movie to such an extent that you can then play around with different variables.

In interviews with Michael Phelps and his coach, they talk so vividly about the mental rehearsal that he goes through. You can't help but conclude that he has reached that stage where he not only mastered the details of that mental movie he's playing, but the door is open to alternative twists in the action he's taking in the movie and possible workarounds. It's really important to tie in Michael Phelps' mental rehearsal with the elements involved in movie watching, so you can unlock the full power of the mental movie method to whatever project you're handling.

THE "SECRET" TO THE MENTAL MOVIE METHOD

The secret to the mental movie method, if it isn't obvious already, is that it is all about rehearsing what you're going to do in your mind. You repeat this over and over again. When you do this, you are not just daydreaming. You're not just imagining stuff that has a very little effect on your waking reality.

Instead, you're tapping the power of your unconscious mind. You are programming your unconscious to align itself with the reality you choose. I can't emphasize this enough. You chose the reality because you popped in a specific movie with precise actions and scenes. It all begins with your choice. You are in control of what goes on in that movie.

Now when you play that movie over and over in your mind, your unconscious is triggered. It starts aligning itself with the reality you choose. You start developing an ideal of how you're supposed to perform for peak results; then, you build up the script in your mind.

Now what makes it really effective is you're not just sticking to some sort of magic bullet "ideal framework" for success. Instead, this is just the starting point; because, the more you watch the mental movie, the more you could anticipate what could go wrong. You do this very quickly. If you keep playing the movie repeatedly, you figure out what you should do to achieve great results. You know how you should respond when things go wrong or unanticipated events pop up.

You develop an advanced view of what could go wrong and how you can respond to them optimally. You can achieve peak results by simply repeating this process over and over again in your head. The keyword here is optimal. The great thing about this approach is you're in complete control. You don't actually have to act it out at that particular point in time. Instead, you play this in your head again and again. When it comes to practicing, you go through the script and align your physical actions with the moves that you've rehearsed in your head.

What makes this approach so powerful?

First of all, you can do it anywhere. It is very portable. You don't have to be at a specific place. You can sit back and relax at a café, close your eyes and think about what you're going to do for the project that you're working on.

You can do this right before you go to bed, before you practice, or right after.

Another thing that is awesome about this method is that it helps you achieve an emotional state of calm. This is really important because when unexpected twists and turns show up, it's too easy to get thrown off track and get frazzled. Unfortunately, when you get thrown off by the unanticipated, a lot of your sense of control goes out the window. You then, become desperate; in many cases, you forget the script, and you start struggling.

This is where a lot of otherwise highly prepared and supremely talented athletes and performers get it wrong. They keep training, but their training doesn't prepare them for the emotional impact of unexpected events. Accordingly, they start to panic and their performance suffers as a result.

By using the mental movie method and mastering it, your actions "play out" in front of you, and you maintain a tremendous sense of control. It's like you're watching and acting out the movie at the same time. This enables you to take action while having a model with which to compare your present action to. On top of all this, you are able to anticipate problems, and you have a plan already locked in so you can work around whatever issues materialize.

61

HOW TO BENEFIT FROM THE MENTAL MOVIE METHOD

So what are the benefits of the mental movie method, if I have not been clear already in the previous chapter. It's really important for you to understand how the mental movie benefits you so you can put in the time to make it work for you. I don't mean to give you any illusions, but it takes work. It takes consistent practice for this to pay off.

If you're still unclear whether it's effective or not, just look up Michael Phelps' statistics and amazing record of victory. You should get all the proof you need. If that isn't awesome enough, always remember that he's not alone. There are lots of other people who are at the top of their field in many industries, fields of specialization, and walks of life which also use the mental movie method. Whether they use it to achieve physical fitness, or increase productivity and enhance work quality, the method works for them. If it works for them, it can work for you too.

Here are just some of the benefits of this method. I'm not going to claim that this is the comprehensive list of all the benefits this technique is capable of bringing into your life, but this should give you a fairly clear idea of why you should try it. Not tomorrow, not next week, but today.

Remain calm and in control

It's too easy to lose when you are just running like a chicken with its head cut off. You have to remain calm and in control. Even if things seem to be going off track or falling apart, when you choose to remain calm and in control, you increase the likelihood that you will identify the workaround and adopt it. In other words, you would be able to get out from under the problem. What could have been a disaster might actually end up working in your favor because your competitors got thrown off track. You're the one who remained calm and in control; you made it all the way through the finish line.

Get a clear idea of how you're supposed to perform at the right time

As I keep mentioning repeatedly in this book at the risk of sounding like a broken record, one of the main reasons why people fail to achieve predictable and sustainable success is they lose sight of the fact that their performance matters only at a specific time and place. You can't just apply some sort of blanket technique that may only be optimal for certain settings. It doesn't work that way. When you use the mental movie method, you get a clear idea of how you're supposed to perform at that specific time. You get a template, and you layer on all the things that can throw you off so that you operate at your peak level performance.

Achieve autopilot success

Since you mentally rehearsed what you will be doing, success becomes more automatic and predictable. You already have a script. All your preparations are aligned with the script and contingencies.

Anticipate and respond ideally to things that may throw you off

When certain situations happen that cause people to panic, that's actually an opportunity. Instead of looking at these situations as problems, look at them as opportunities. As I've mentioned before, if you're able to keep calm and minimize your failure while everybody else fails big time, you come out ahead. Competition by definition is comparative.

Do yourself a big favor and keep playing that mental movie in your head so you can see what could go wrong, and you can also spot your options in dealing with them.

The more you play the movie, the more it becomes clear to you that there are certain things you can do that would lead to even better results, or are the ideal courses of action when things happen in your situation.

Keep focused on the big picture

When you go playing your mental movie, there's always an ending. The ending is all too predictable: you win the prize. This ending is not just there as a placeholder. You don't put the ending there because there's nothing left for you to do. The ending gives you a big picture.

Why are you competing? Why are you going through with all this hassle? Why are you putting in the work? The conclusion keeps you focused on the big picture which is the prize at the end of the tunnel.

Conserve your energy and focus only on what's needed for success in your context

This is one benefit that many people would get really excited about. When you play the mental movie repeatedly, you achieve a state of calm and confidence regarding what you're going to do. This doesn't mean that you're going to stop training or trying. What it does mean is that you would be able to see the project or competition in its proper context, and you would be confident enough that you can conserve your energy and focus only on what's needed for success in that particular context.

This is a lifesaver because the way most people "prepare" is simply to stretch themselves too thin. The example about the bar exam actually plays out time and again. If you ask people who flunked the bar exam and had to take it twice, thrice, or even five times, a lot of them would tell you that topics and subjects they didn't concentrate on showed up in the test. When you would be able to achieve a state of calm where you can conserve your energy, look at the context of what's going on, and focus on what's needed to win or achieve in a particular situation.

Activate and preserve your sense of urgency

When you play the mental movie method, you achieve a state of calm, but you are also able to control your sense of urgency. You know what to expect, and when you are in the middle of the competition, you could unleash your sense of urgency but in a calm way. You don't panic; you're not frantic. You don't expend unnecessary emotional and physical energy. By being more focused and concentrated, you increase the likelihood of success.

Be Grateful Ahead of Time

One of the biggest secrets that I can share is to act as if your goal has already been accomplished. You will trick your subconscious mind into believing that you are the type of person that is capable of achieving this goal, so it will become activated and start looking for opportunities to help you achieve it. You also should be thankful for achieving your goal BEFORE you have actually achieved it. This is another way to convince your mind that you deserve and have achieved your goal. When you are grateful, you make your mind open, receptive, and positive, allowing your subconscious to take over and look for the right skills, opportunities, and people to help you achieve your goal.

5 STEPS TO CREATING THE PERFECT MENTAL MOVIE

To recap; the mental movie method can help you be more successful in all areas of your life. I'm not just talking about sports or any non-sport competition. While it will definitely help you in those types of competition, you can use this method for all areas of your life. We're talking about better relationships, losing weight, feeling better about yourself, and otherwise living your life to its fullest potential. If you're feeling stuck or feeling like you're not achieving the kind of success that you deserve, then you need to pay close attention to the mental movie method.

Another point that I need you to direct your attention to is the fact that this mental movie method is slightly different from the public pronouncements of Michael Phelps and his coach regarding how they use mental rehearsal. While it does share many common features, it is an improvement on the pronouncements they make regarding the method that they use.

Now, I'm not sure why they did not cover certain points; maybe it's for competitive reasons. Maybe they don't want to share the "secret sauce" to their system, and they just want to describe a general approach. Whatever the case may be; what you will be getting in the five steps I'm going to highlight below is the complete mental movie method. This approach to achieving personal success enables you to perform at a very high level of quality and productivity, and it also enables you to anticipate problems.

We live in an imperfect world. You shouldn't need me to tell you that. You should have already figured that on your own. There are all sorts of things that can happen even if you have the best-laid plans. After all, according to the old saying, "Life is what happens to you while you're busy making other plans." That's just the way life works.

Accordingly, if you were just to use the mental movie method mentioned by Michael Phelps and other people who practice success mental rehearsal, you may fall short. That's not enough. There is still one key component that is left out. This key component answers the fundamental question of: What do you do when things fall apart? Regardless of how excited you are or how well you prepare to do a good job; things can and do happen, which will jeopardize your best-laid plans. You must get ready for these unforeseen situations.

The mental movie method has five steps. Each of these steps has essential parts that you need to pay close attention to. Make sure that you take each step and master them. Do not jump from one step to another and race through them. That's not going to work. You must master, understand, and be comfortable with it. Once you reach that high level of comfort, then you move on to the next step. Otherwise, you might be settling for a tiny fraction of the success that you could achieve with this amazing personal success process. Let's begin.

Step #1 Understand the task you're going to do

I need you to go over that sentence again. Understand the task you're going to do. This seems quite obvious. It would seem fairly intuitive, but you shouldn't go with your assumptions. Understanding the task you're going to do doesn't mean you assume that just because this task looks like previous tasks or competitions then you know everything already. What this means is it has to be at a specific time, process, and place. That competition, that you're going to participate in, is very different from all the other competitions before it and after it.

I need you to think along these lines. You can't just coast on what you've done in the past. You can't proceed based on what you know from your previous tasks, competitions, or projects. That falls short; you have to understand this specific task you're going to do.

Accordingly, you should research your competition. Who are you up against? What do they do? How have they performed in the past? What are their strengths and weaknesses? Next, you should research the venue. Where is the presentation going to take place? Where are you going to meet that member of the opposite sex? What do you know about the venue? How do people perform in the venue? What are contingencies that might come up at the venue?

The next thing that you should do is to research the process. Now that you have a clear idea of what the task is, what processes are involved? What are the most obvious processes and which are the ones that are less obvious? Finally, focus on the specifics of everything that you're going to be doing. The more specific your understanding, the clearer the picture will be in your mind when you run the mental movie. Also, when you're clear on all the specifics, the script that you're going to play over and over in your mind is going to be truly relevant to the project, competition, or obstacle you're going to be dealing with.

Step #2 Understand contingencies

In my opinion, this is the secret sauce. A lot of the public pronouncements of people who say they use mental rehearsal techniques often leave this out. From my own experiences, as well as observations, I believe that this is the secret sauce. This is what will put you over the top. The mental movie method is powerful enough if you're just going to use it for a mental rehearsal. It can get you 99% of the way there, but if you truly want to stand head and shoulders over the rest, you need to understand contingencies. Put simply, these are things that could go wrong.

Now you don't need me to remind you that all sorts of things go wrong. It doesn't matter how well you plan, how motivated you are, or what your attitude is. Ultimately, it doesn't matter; it just happens. So instead of beating yourself up and feeling really bad because something unforeseen happened and moping around like it's all unfair, it's time to get real.

First, you need to understand that stuff does happen. Once we've stopped denying that then we need to look at all the possible contingencies that could happen. Keep in mind that possible doesn't necessarily mean that it is probable. It's possible that you can walk outside your house, and somebody will throw a bag at you and inside is 10-million dollars. Anything is possible, but is it likely? Probably not, so it's really important to go through this step by first focusing on what is possible. Get a clear idea of all the things that could go wrong with that specific task you're going to do.

Now, the next thing you need to do is to sort them into two bags or baskets: probable and not so probable. This is where things get real. What are the things that could happen that are more likely to happen? This doesn't mean that they will happen; they're just more likely to happen. Sort those in the probable basket; everything else goes in the improbable basket. You should put more focus, attention, and time into studying probable contingencies.

After you've done that, and you've gone over this list several times, the next step is to sort them again into three categories: neutral complications, positive complications, and negative complications. It's important to do this sorting because this categorization impacts the course of actions you're going to be taking.

After you've done the sorting, ask yourself, "If neutral complications materialize, what do I do? What is the workaround? How do I deal with this?" Keep analyzing this until your actions make sense to you. Obviously, when neutral complications occur, your main focus should be not getting thrown off and to avoid distraction.

The same applies to negative complications. Got through your list and imagine what are the things that can go wrong and will throw me off. This is not a question of maybe, but will. These events would have a really negative effect on my performance and my ability to achieve the success that I'm looking for.

After you've done that, you then, ask yourself, "What are the things I could do to work around these problems, avoid them, get out from under them, or deal with them, so I don't get thrown off my game?" This will take a bit more work because this will require you to be quite imaginative. It will test your creativity. The good news is if you keep practicing this, things will be clear eventually.

Finally, prepare for positive contingencies. These are positive complications that work to help you. For example, if a competitor breaks a leg or someone who is thinking of investing in your company just sold one of his companies for a billion dollars. How do you maximize the opportunities presented by positive contingencies? Focus on that question. Again, keep coming up with solutions so that when opportunities and challenges appear, while you are in the middle of tasks, you are not thrown off.

Just as importantly, when opportunities appear, you take advantage of them optimally. You don't just stand around with your jaw on the ground and babble to yourself, and fail to take advantage. Competitors who win over and over again have developed a skill for spotting opportunities a mile away. Once they spot the opportunity, everything else kicks into gear; they know what to say at the right time to the right people to produce results. You can do the same.

Similarly, when the worst situations happen, you can just let it slide off your back. You keep pushing forward, and you achieve victory. This is how you come up against superior competition. I need you to understand that. I need you to wrap your mind around that concept, because a lot of people get intimidated.

When they look at their competition, and they see how big, strong, well-funded, well-prepared, and educated the competition is, they just drivel up and die inside. They put up a good game. When it comes to appearances, they look like they got their game together, but deep inside, they're scared. So it's really important to avoid that mental state because it doesn't help you. You have to deal with contingencies effectively. Follow the tips in this section very closely, and you will get the "secret sauce" you need to come out on top.

Step #3 Setting up your mental video

Now that you've gone through steps 1 and 2, fully understood and mastered them, the next step is you set up your mental video. First of all, you set up an ideal situation in your mind. The ideal situation is just as Michael Phelps says regarding his mental rehearsals. This is where everything is ideal. Everything is as expected. The right people are there; the right context is there, and you're doing the right things. This is your base script.

As I've mentioned previously, we are going to take your base script, and then we're going to make permutations, so we can effectively handle contingencies. However, you need to lay the base first. This is your base script. It involves the ideal situation; set it up in your mind. The best way to do this though is to write it down first and keep going through what you've written then simplifying things, shortening things, or otherwise, taking out the clutter.

Once everything is clear, compact, and easy to understand, then you keep repeating it until you memorize it. Once you've memorized it, you should have enough to visualize. By visualization, I am talking about fully immersing yourself in the ideal situation in your mind. It first starts with your sense of vision. You imagine things that you will see. You

imagine the scene, details of all the elements in the scene, and the action. It all involves what you see.

Now, after you've done the visualization on an optical level, the next step is to visualize in 3D. This means paying attention to what you'd hear, smell, taste, and touch. Why go this extra step? The more all your senses are engaged, the more realistic the visualized mental scene becomes. Eventually, you reach the point that you need where you feel that you're actually in the visualization.

This is where things become real. Why? We could all talk a big game about why we need to lose weight. It's very easy to accept the fact that, "Hey; I'm overweight," intellectually. However, the problem is, that just takes place on the intellectual level. It doesn't become real enough for me to hit the gym, go on a diet, watch what I eat, buy the right products to boost my weight loss, unless I feel it in my heart.

Without emotional urgency, all these things that I realize I should be doing remain safely compartmentalized in some filing cabinet in my mind. When you use visualization, it's not enough to "see" things, you also have to use all your other senses so your emotional state is triggered. When you become emotionally engaged, it becomes real enough for your mind to keep repeating it again and again until your actions align with it.

You focus on how you feel, on how you respond in that particular situation, and most importantly; you imagine the victory. Imagine how it would feel to cross that finish line. Imagine how it would feel to get that race that added another $100,000 dollars to your annual income. Imagine how it would feel to have that medal on you. Whatever you are trying to achieve, just imagine that endpoint where all the sweat, tears, time, and effort that you put in finally paid off. Allow yourself to feel it.

This may seem funny and strange, but a lot of people can't get to this point. Why? They get the idea that they should compete. They get the idea that they should work towards a promotion or a great job. The problem is, they focus primarily on their needs. They focus on getting from one day to the next. That's not enough. You're basically just operating out of fear and necessity; you have to operate out of love.

I am, of course, talking about pro-activity. You desire an outcome. Unless that love is there, it's too easy for your mind to make up all sorts of excuses and justifications that ultimately enable you to rob yourself of victory. This happens all the time. So, allow yourself not just to imagine the victory in terms of intellectual details, but also imagine the emotional impact of that victory.

How it would feel. How it would impact you as a person on many different levels. How it would impact your self-confidence and self-esteem. How it would impact how you think other people view you. These all flow together, and they enable you to feel a tremendous surge of urgency so you can do whatever and however long it takes to achieve that success. Get hooked on that feeling.

This ultimately enables you to remember what you need to do to win in this particular context. Again, it's all contextual. You need to go through this step #3's complete process, so you have what it takes to use your base mental video to deliver victory.

Step #4 Setting up a foolproof mental video

Now, with Step #3, with everything else being equal, you should have enough to succeed. You should have enough set up to win again and again. However, we live in reality. In reality, people fall through. People don't keep their promises. Nature is fickle. Money gets lost. Political intrigues and backstabbing occur. All sorts of things can go wrong; that's just the kind of world we live in.

Accordingly, your mental video should factor this all in. These are the steps you need to take. First, you need to visualize everything happening in an ideal setting. In an ideal world, what would victory look like? What would you be doing? What would your competitors be doing? How is everything set up? This is your base; this is your starting point.

Now, the next step is to go back to the contingencies you mastered in Step #2 and visualize them appearing. Ideally, you should visualize them one by one. After you mastered handling one particular problem, you should move on to the next. Keep going down your list and use the mental rehearsal method. When you do this, you prime yourself to cope with less than ideal settings. This is, again, at the risk of sounding like a broken record, the core of the mental movie method.

Because anybody can do the method involving ideal settings. Anybody can daydream that everything is going to be fine, but that's not how it works. That's why a lot of people, regardless of how well-prepared and trained they are, end up getting crushed. So, you have to cope with less than ideal settings. Running these less than ideal scenarios in your mind repeatedly, you figure out the most optimal way to deal with them if they appear. You become familiarized with these alternative scenes. At the end, it's still the same; you still win.

So, what is the net effect of this approach? When you visualize less than ideal situations and how you victoriously deal with them over and over again, you become at ease with your base script getting thrown off. This is your goal. You want to feel at ease. You want to achieve that sense of emotional control. You should imagine the location, the details of the complication, and contingencies involved.

Similarly, you should also imagine social challenges. Imagine the people who are going to be there. What if they're jerks? What if they're very mean to you? What if they try to make your life hell? Keep going through these alternative scenarios with the aim of developing a feeling of ease. When you feel comfortable, you can take action that would produce more optimal results.

It goes without saying that you should visualize yourself overcoming all these contingencies. Imagine things falling apart, and there you are, acting in an optimal way. Now we're not just talking about seeing a scene where things are falling apart and then you fast-forward to you, with your arms raised in victory. No, that doesn't work; you actually have to go visualize the scene of you dealing with the things that have gone wrong. This requires specific mental rehearsal with precise details. Otherwise, step #4 is not working for you. This is a test of your creativity, imagination, and resilience.

Step #5 Fill in all the details

This may seem a bit redundant because I've already mentioned this in Step #3. However, it requires its own section so you do not forget it. It also requires its own section because the emotional engagement required by the mental movie method is paramount. Without emotional engagement, you're going to fall apart. This section also covers the importance of constantly repeating the mental movie method and optimizing it.

First, you need to make sure that you visualize in three dimensions. Don't just focus on sights and appearances, focus on sounds, scents, tastes and textures also. The more you do this, the more you become emotionally engaged. As I keep repeating, emotional urgency is required to wake up your unconscious.

The real hero here is your unconscious. You're taking the limited consciousness that you have to wake up your inner giant, which is your unconscious. If you feel limited in your ability to turn your ideas into reality, it's because your conscious state is limited. Believe it or not, your unconscious state is unlimited.

So, when you get your unconscious state emotionally engaged, you wake up its power, and your ability to turn hopes, wishes, dreams, and ideas into reality explodes. If you keep it up, you become unstoppable. Again, emotional engagement involves asking yourself, "How would I feel in that specific space and time?" Keep it as detailed as possible.

It's important to repeat the process continuously. Don't just go through the mental movie once or twice right before the competition or sales presentation; it doesn't work that way. You have to keep repeating this in your mind until you achieve a sense of mastery and ease. You have to feel comfortable. When you're repeating your vision, you should not just go through the motions. You should work on maximizing the details. Make sure that there are no sights, sounds, scents, tastes, and textures that you overlooked.

When do you know that you have repeated enough? It's very simple. You have memorized details. That's how much you should repeat the mental movie in your head. Moreover, when you repeat the movie in a loop, you end up speeding the visualization. First, you master the details, then you focus on the time. Everything is still detailed, but you can notice all of them in a relatively short period of time.

When you keep repeating this along with the contingencies, your overall time frame is reduced. In addition, the sense of mastery and comfort you feel is increased. By the time you go on that date, apply for that job or promotion, or take that test, you are very confident. Finally, you should also pair your visualization with skill building and preparation.

The mental movie method is not going to work for you if you do not physically take action on it. Like I said earlier, I can imagine myself going to the gym, bench pressing 300 pounds, running around the track field, and swimming 100 laps a day in the pool, and nothing will happen if I'm just sitting here in my chair, drinking beer, and eating Cheetos. You have to pair your visualization with skill building and preparation.

Normally, this is not a big deal because people who look into mental rehearsal techniques are already doing physical training. They're already doing job training and skill building. They just need a competitive edge. **Still, it would be irresponsible of me if I did not point this out, because there are people out there who have a mistaken understanding of the law of attraction.** They think that the law of attraction, properly understood, is only about thinking the right thoughts.

No, that's a big part, but you're missing other pieces of the puzzle.

There has to be action and actual work involved. Continue working on your skills and prepare. Your training is just a piece of the puzzle, but the visualization component puts it all together. A good analogy would be the mental movie method is the cement that puts the bricks of training, skill, and context together.

USING YOUR MENTAL MOVIE TO ACHIEVE MOMENTUM

The more you practice, the clearer your vision should get. It becomes easier and easier for you. It also becomes much faster. You need to do this over and over again, because you want to achieve that emotional state of ease. Things that used to intimidate, scare, and discourage you no longer have that effect. Everything becomes not just more doable, but probable. I need to emphasize that. We're not just talking about "how I can do it," it's "I will do it" or "I am very likely to do it."

Do you see how this works? Because anybody can say I can do it. I can do it as a statement of possibility. As I've mentioned in previous chapters, everything is possible. We're not just talking about possibility here, but probability. The mental movie method, if implemented correctly, makes success and victory probable; not just possible, but very likely to happen.

You need to wrap your mind around that. You need to focus on that. That's what you're trying to do. You're trying to make success, which you've found so frustrating before, not just possible, but likely to happen. One important technique you can use to reach that stage is to create an upward spiral. Use the mental movie method in a small task. See it in action; enjoy its benefits. This is your "proof of concept."

You keep repeating this for small, easier tasks. Once it becomes clear to you that this method works, it will be obvious that when you visualize reality, it happens. You need to reach that stage, because the more your actual experience fits your visualized reality, the more motivated you become to try and try it again. Not just try it on the small stuff, but start scaling it up until you tackle bigger and bigger projects. You start to slay greater giants in your life. Eventually, everything lines up between your inner world and outer world.

The reason why so many people struggle through life and feel they're stuck in a life of mediocrity or even failure is because their inner world doesn't line up with their outer world. They think all these great things in their imagination. They have all these hopes and dreams, but their outer world doesn't line up because they don't prepare the right way. There is no connection.

Interestingly enough, a lot of those people who are frustrated are objectively well-trained and have a lot of skills. The problem is they do not use the mental movie method or any inner reality shaping system as cement to hold all the different pieces of their lives together. Now, this doesn't mean they're complete losers, and they fail all the time. They do achieve victory from time to time, but if you were serious in achieving victory over and over again on a predictable basis, you need to use the mental movie method.

You can shape your reality just by thinking of certain things and allowing yourself to be so emotionally engaged based on your thoughts; you take action to change your reality. I can't emphasize that point enough. The truth is, the world couldn't care less about what you're thinking, feeling, or getting motivated by. Really, all of that is happening in your head. However, the world sits up and pays attention when you take action. That's right; the world only cares about objective reality.

Objective reality is all about action. It's all about how we change our environment, but the good news is that it all begins with what we consciously think. That's how we shape our reality. And wait, it gets even better. If this whole process of changing our external reality all starts with what we think, then this means, we're always in control. We may not be able to control all the things that are happening around us. We definitely can't control Mother Nature; however, we can control what we think and focus on.

Use visualization to master your personal reality. It doesn't matter whether you're competing in sports, trying to get a great job or get promoted. It doesn't matter whether you're trying to meet the right person for you, or you're trying to hit the gym and develop a body that you want. Visualization applies to all areas of your life. Use the mental movie method to unlock your inner champion.

SAMPLE MENTAL MOVIE SCRIPT

One of the best self-help books of all time is Psycho-Cybernetics written by Dr. Maxwell Maltz in the 1960's. He was a plastic surgeon that noticed patients who have had their limbs amputated still felt pain that limb.

Even though it had been amputated.

This got him thinking about self-image. He concluded that we become what we think about. He's not the first one to say this, but it really resonated with me.

The whole point of his book is that your mind is like a "heat seeking missile" If it has a goal, infused with emotion and passion, it will figure out how to accomplish it.

There will be trial and error, but if you keep believing in your goal and take action, you will eventually achieve it. He gives the example of a baby reaching for an object on a table. When he first reaches for it, he might miss it, but he will eventually get it.

So belief creates a positive self-image. When you create a positive self-image of yourself ALREADY having accomplished your goal, you will have the motivation and drive to figure it out.

Sit back, openly, confidently, and expectantly with your arms at your side and your head leaning back slightly.

Close your eyes and smile ever so slightly with your mouth and jaws loose and relaxed.

Imagine you're sitting on a cruise ship, looking out at a dark sky early in the morning. The horizon looks purple and is almost glowing. As you sit there, imagine a warm golden rain falling gently on your body.

Enjoy the beautiful peace, and warmth, and serenity of this powerful scene.

For money tell yourself:

- I am *making XXXX dollars per day/week/month/year*

- *I am seeing and feeling this money coming to me*

- *I make this money passively, progressively, consistently, and easily*

- *I am earning this money by helping other people —
I am receiving this money from unexpected sources*

- *For love tell yourself:*

- *I am in a beautiful relationship with someone who I love and who loves me*

- *I am in a happy, supportive relationship*

- *I love my spouse. We are intimate, supportive, and feel like we're on the same team.* I am happy and grateful to have him/her in my life

For health tell yourself:

- *I am healthy and active. I eat a healthy, nutritious diet and enjoy being active. I take care of my body everyday and give it exercise and rest.*

- *My body is healing itself and constantly getting better. I am calm and* grateful that God created me and has given me my body and life.

Now imagine the goal that you seek to achieve. **Imagine yourself already having achieved it. Speak as if you've already achieved it.**

Imagine the power, and confidence, and excitement, and enthusiasm, and gratitude you would feel once you're accomplished it.

KNOW in your mind that you've already achieved it.

That you already have it.

Feel those feelings.

Think those thoughts.

Know that this is the secret to achieving your goals is **to be thankful for already having achieved them.**

Feel it.

Believe it.

Expect it.

Doing this meditation for 5 minutes every day will mold your subconscious mind to expect that reality. It will sharpen your focus, enhance your motivation, and help guide you to the actions and activities that you need to take to achieve them.

It's incredibly powerful.

Now go do it and enjoy the feelings of pride, confidence, gratitude, and excitement that come with it.

1. **So choose a goal.**

2. **Imagine, visualize, and see yourself having already achieved it.**

3. **Sense the amazing feelings of achieving your goal.**

THE JACK CANFIELD MENTAL MOVIE SCRIPT

Go through the following three steps:

STEP 1. Imagine sitting in a movie theater, the lights dim, and then the movie starts. It is a movie of you doing perfectly whatever it is that you want to do better. See as much detail as you can create, including your clothing, the expression on your face, small body movements, the environment and any other people that might be around. Add in any sounds you would be hearing — traffic, music, other people talking, cheering. And finally, recreate in your body any feelings you think you would be experiencing as you engage in this activity.

STEP 2. Get out of your chair, walk up to the screen, open a door in the screen and enter into the movie. Now experience the whole thing again from inside of yourself, looking out through your eyes. This is called an "embodied image" rather than a "distant image." It will deepen the impact of the experience. Again, see everything in vivid detail, hear the sounds you would hear, and feel the feelings you would feel.

STEP 3. Finally, walk back out of the screen that is still showing the picture of you performing perfectly, return to your seat in the theater, reach out and grab the screen and shrink it down to the size of a cracker. Then, bring this miniature screen up to your mouth, chew it up and swallow it. Imagine that each tiny piece — just like a hologram — contains the full picture of you performing well. Imagine all these little screens traveling down into your stomach and out through the bloodstream into every cell of your body. Then imagine that every cell of your body is lit up with a movie of you performing perfectly. It's like one of those appliance store windows where 50 televisions are all tuned to the same channel.

When you have finished this process — it should take less than five minutes — you can open your eyes and go about your business. If you make this part of your daily routine, you will be amazed at how much improvement you will see in your life.

Use Affirmations to Support Your Visualization

An affirmation is a statement that evokes not only a picture, but the experience of already having what you want. Here's an example of an affirmation:

I am happily vacationing 2 months out of the year in a tropical paradise, and working just four days a week owning my own business.

Repeating an affirmation several times a day keeps you focused on your goal, strengthens your motivation, and programs your subconscious by sending an order to your crew to do whatever it takes to make that goal happen.

Expect Results

Through writing down your goals, using the power of visualization and repeating your affirmations, you can achieve **amazing results**.

Visualization and affirmations allow you to **change your beliefs**, **assumptions**, and **opinions** about the most important person in your life — YOU! They allow you to harness the 18 billion brain cells in your brain and get them all working in a singular and purposeful direction.

Your subconscious will become engaged in a process that transforms you forever. The process is invisible and doesn't take a long time.

DON'T FORGET YOUR FREE GIFTS

Get Your FREE Gift #1

Get my 1-page cheat sheet **"60 Seconds of Focus"**

I will show you how to develop **ruthless focus** so you can:

- SKYROCKET your productivity
- TURBOCHARGE your income
- BOOST your self-confidence
- ANNIHILATE debt

My 1-page cheat sheet will help you do all of this by harnessing the power of **ruthless focus.**

Click the link below to get your free gift:

http://www.5xYourFocus.com

Get Your FREE Gift #2

I will also email you my other super-popular videos I use to visualize my goals and get focused:

- **6 Minute Daily Visualization for Goal Achievement**

- **How to Manifest Your Desires (very powerful visualization)**

-

It takes less than 20 minutes to go through and will help you get focused and prime your subconscious mind for success.

You can get access to all of that AND my "**60 Seconds of Focus**" cheat sheet by going here:

www.5xYourFocus.com

Please Leave a Review

I hope you enjoyed this book. If you did, please leave me a review. It will only take 30 seconds and it would mean a LOT to me as an author.

We live and die by reviews.

- They help us know how our readers feel about our work

- They give us the motivation to keep writing

- They help others learn about our books

So please leave a review now.

Thanks in advance ☺

www.ingramcontent.com/pod-product-compliance
Lightning Source LLC
Chambersburg PA
CBHW031143250726
48655CB00002B/806